I0429598

Yoga for Beginners: The Best Yoga Poses and Techniques for 6-Pack Abs

All rights Reserved. No part of this publication or the information in it may be quoted from or reproduced in any form by means such as printing, scanning, photocopying or otherwise without prior written permission of the copyright holder.

Disclaimer and Terms of Use: Effort has been made to ensure that the information in this book is accurate and complete, however, the author and the publisher do not warrant the accuracy of the information, text and graphics contained within the book due to the rapidly changing nature of science, research, known and unknown facts and internet. The Author and the publisher do not hold any responsibility for errors, omissions or contrary interpretation of the subject matter herein. This book is presented solely for motivational and informational purposes only.

Table of Contents

Introduction

Building a strong body is the basis of health and fitness. A person who doesn't have a fit body finds it hard to maintain his mental fitness too. In the recent years, the trend of having a muscular physique and 6-pack abs has become a parameter of fitness for most men. Although this is not entirely true, it has become a trend that most of the youngsters like to follow as a challenge. They want to prove that they are strong enough to achieve it. However, getting 6-pack abs is not that easy for everyone. Some people have an athletic figure which makes it easy for them to get a 6-pack abs. But some men are not so fortunate. They need to build an athletic body in order to get a muscular body. In this review we will be discussing about Yoga and how it can help in sculpting a 6-pack abs.

Benefits Of Yoga

Yoga is an ancient art that was developed several thousand years ago. It is native to the land of India. Few decades ago, it was introduced to the western world and since then it has been popularized by different types of fitness centres and fitness gurus. If you wish to begin with Yoga, it is important to understand the role and benefits of Yoga. In order to practice yoga, one needs to lead a disciplined life. Hence, it is imperative to understand the rules and regulations required for practicing yoga.

1. Yoga is different from other types of exercises. In Yoga there are different poses that have different meanings. Attaining these poses and retaining them is the goal of yoga. In doing so the practitioner gets lots of energy and he ends up stretching his muscles in different ways. Just by attaining various poses as Asanas he gets lot of benefits. It is like a treatment rather than an exercise.

2. Yoga primarily helps in building a disease-free body. This is the first goal of yoga. Secondly, it makes the body strong and immune to diseases. Thirdly, it makes the body quite strong and athletic.

3. Yoga makes us more flexible. If you are practicing yoga, you will be developing a flexible body as well as mind. This will eventually help you in sculpting a muscular physique. Yoga can help your body in building lean muscle mass. This will make it easier for you to attain your goal of 6-pack abs.

4. Yoga is quite beneficial in developing strength and freshness. When other exercises generate fatigue, yoga energizes a person's body. After a session of yoga, the practitioners feel very lively and full of energy. Hence, many people practice yoga along with other activities like weight training, cardio, swimming, jogging etc. Yoga helps them in replenishing their body with a steady flow of energy.

5. Yoga strengthens the nervous system and helps in faster physical development. If you are practicing yoga with other exercises, you will get faster results. Hence, if you practice weight training along with yoga, you will be getting better results from your weight training. This will help you in building a 6-pack abs without much delay.

6. Yoga helps in mental development. Regular practitioners of yoga derive lot of mental calm and

steadiness. Yoga also helps in improving the concentration power of your mind. This can indirectly help you in focusing on other forms of exercises and workouts. Even if the results are slow, yoga will encourage your mind to focus on your goals.

7. Yoga improves the oxygen supply in our body. Practicing yoga helps our body to make optimum utilization of oxygen received by our cells. This in turn helps in better absorption of food and nutrients. Thus it helps the body in deriving faster results from various types of exercises.

8. Yoga improves blood circulation. Blood circulation is one of the major factors that make us more energetic. By improving blood circulation, yoga helps the body in better absorption of food and oxygen. This eventually helps in overall development of muscles. Thus yoga can help you in attaining your goal of 6-pack abs.

9. There are several poses in Yoga that focuses on the strengthening of abdomen. These poses help in fat burning and muscle development. By practicing

these poses you can improve your chances of building a 6-pack abs.

10. In order to get a 6-pack abs, you need to work out on a regular basis. You need to do certain special weight training programs that can drain your patience and will power. However, if you are practicing yoga you will be able to maintain your efforts. Yoga helps in developing patience and it makes the body strong enough to endure hours of workout sessions.

11. Diet is an important aspect when it comes to bodybuilding and weight training. You need to have a special protein-rich diet for getting a well-shaped and muscular body. Yoga practice can aid the body in absorbing all the nutrients provided by you. It helps the body in making optimum use of all the resources. This in turn can help you in shaping a muscular physique.

12. Weight training and special workouts meant for abs can exhaust your body as well as mind. Nonetheless, yoga can help you in relieving all the stress and exhaustion. Thus it can help you in relaxing your muscles.

How To Begin With Yoga?

1. In order to begin with yoga, you need to find a good yoga master. You can join a yoga class in your locality or find a good yoga trainer in your town. You cannot learn yoga on your own.

2. There are some people who try to practice yoga on their own. They try to follow the instructions given in a book or an online tutorial. Although, there is nothing wrong in practicing yoga at your home, experts recommend to find a good teacher who can monitor your practices. Yoga is a very powerful tool and if it is wrongly practiced, it can lead to severe consequences. Hence, it is safer to find a yoga guru or master who can guide you personally.

3. When you are beginning with yoga, you need to mention your goals. If you wish to practice yoga for getting a 6-pack abs, you need to perform special poses that can help you to strengthen your abdominal muscles. Hence, you should discuss with your yoga teacher about your requirements so that he or she can guide you accordingly.

4. It is better to practice yoga during the morning hours. Although you can practice it at anytime, there are certain rules to be followed. You should practice yoga on an empty stomach. However, you can consume some liquid food before your practice session. If you are practicing yoga in the evening, make sure that you eat something around 4 hours before your yoga session. In 4 hours your body will digest the food and leave your stomach empty.

5. You should avoid eating for 1 hour after the conclusion of your yoga session. Following such rules are quite essential to derive the right kind of benefits from your yoga practice.

6. Yoga is also a spiritual exercise. Hence, it is important to keep your mind focussed while performing yoga. There is no point in doing yoga when you are stressed or depressed.

7. In yoga, certain poses need to be performed together. Even if your aim is to practice yoga poses that enhances your stomach muscles, you need to do certain additional poses that are essential to balance the effects of certain poses. Similarly, you need to do certain poses in a specific order. This is to

counteract the effects created by certain yoga steps. For deriving the right kind of benefits it is essential to follow such steps.

8. It is essential to find a yoga teacher or master who has a great deal of knowledge about yoga and its effects on human body and mind. Find a certified teacher who has a good deal of experience in training lot of students.

9. Since your goal is to develop a 6-pack abs, you need a yoga teacher who has some good knowledge about weight training and bodybuilding. He should be able to advise you on various ways to bring a balance between your bodybuilding efforts and your yoga training.

10. Once you begin with your yoga sessions you need to continue them on a regular basis. If you quit in between or if you are irregular, then you may not derive the desired results.

Different Yoga Poses

In yoga a pose is known as an Asana. There are many Asanas in yoga and you need to practices only a few among them. One of the most important exercises in yoga is known as the Sun Salutation or the Surya Namaskara. It is a series of different poses that blend into each other forming an elaborate exercise-like system. Sun salutation is actually performed to please the Sun, who is a deity according to Indian mythology. By doing Sun Salutation one attains several benefits. It helps in curing a number of diseases and it makes the body immune to countless number of diseases.

Sun Salutation consists of a series of steps that help in active weight loss. Practicing this specific yoga exercise on a regular basis can reduce your abdominal fat and help you in getting a 6-pack abs.

Sun Salutation is usually performed at the beginning of a yoga session. Before Sun Salutation, you can do certain warm up exercises that prepare the body for dealing with more workouts. However, the actually yoga begins with Sun Salutation. Explained below are the 12 steps of this special yoga exercise.

Steps In Sun Salutation

1. The First step of Sun Salutation begins with a standing pose with hands joined together as in a prayer.

2. In the next step, you should raise both your arms and bend backwards. Turn your gaze towards the sky. In this pose you will be stretching your abdomen and spine. This helps in strengthening the muscles of your abdomen and also the joints of your spine.

3. In the third step you should bend down and place your hands on the floor on either side of your feet. While bending down you should keep your knees straight. This step helps in reducing the fat around your abdomen. It helps in getting a flat stomach.

4. In the fourth step you should extend your left leg backwards and bend your right leg at the knee. Lower your body with the support of your arms and bend your torso backwards. Turn your gaze towards the sky. This pose helps you in reducing the fat

around your lower abdomen. It helps in strengthening the muscles around your waist and also your back.

5. In the next step you should extend your right leg backwards and turn your torso downwards. Bend your body at the waist level and support your body with both your arms. Right now your entire body would resemble an inverted 'V' shape.

6. Now lower your body and slowly touch your knees on the floor. Your torso should also be touching the floor. But your hips should be in the air. While doing all these steps both your hands should be placed on the floor.

7. In the next step you should raise your torso with the support of your arms. Let your legs press firmly against the floor. Raise your entire upper body right from your stomach. Turn your gaze towards the sky. Stay in this pose for few seconds. This step helps in tightening your stomach muscles. It is also beneficial in reducing your belly fat.

8. From here you should repeat the steps in the earlier poses. Gently lift the body with the support of your arms and again assume the shape of an inverted 'V'.

9. In the next step you should lower your body and move your right leg towards the front and bend it at the knee. Keep your left leg in the same position. Turn your torso backwards and turn your gaze towards the sky.

10. Next, you should slowly move your left leg forward and get up. However, do not raise your torso. You should stand on your feet but bend down and keep your hands on the floor, on either side of your feet.

11. In this step you should slowly raise your arms and torso and come to a standing position. Keep your arms up and bend your torso backwards. Stretch yourself.

12. In the next step you should straighten your back and lower your arms and once again join your hands together as if in a prayer.

These 12 steps complete a single round of Sun Salutation. You can practice this exercise slowly or repeat them rapidly. Both have different benefits. These 12 poses flow from one step to another in a smooth way. They expand and contract the body in a rhythm. You have to practice these yoga steps on a daily basis. They can help you in making your abdominal muscles stronger and tighter. They also provide flexibility to all the joints in your body. Sun Salutation has several benefits. It helps in fighting different types of diseases and makes the body strong and immune. In order to shape your body, it would be beneficial if you perform this exercise in a slow pace. If possible, you may do 12 rounds of Sun Salutation in order to derive maximum benefits from it.

Note that, when you are doing Sun Salutation, you should choose a time before sunset.

How To Prepare For Yoga?

In order to perform yoga, you should make certain preparations. They are as listed below.

1. You should practice yoga on an empty stomach. Morning time is most suitable.

2. You should choose a clean place for doing yoga. Do not change the place often. Keep a fixed place for your daily yoga practice. This will make you more comfortable.

3. There shouldn't be any disturbing noises in the background when you are practicing yoga.

4. Avoid wearing tight clothes while doing yoga. Wear clean clothes that allow maximum movements.

5. Drink water before you begin with your yoga session. This will make your body more flexible.

6. The place you select should receive enough sun light. Do not choose a dark place. Natural illumination is better than artificial light.

7. When you are doing yoga, there should be enough oxygen in the atmosphere. Choose an open place like a balcony or a terrace. If you choose to do it in a room, then select a room that has good ventilation and air supply.

Apart from Sun Salutation there are quite a few yoga poses or Asanas that help in strengthening your abdominal muscles. Practicing them can help you in getting a 6-pack abs without much difficulty.

1. **Leg raises**

- Leg raise is a basic exercise in yoga. It helps in building your abdominal muscles.

- Lie down on your back and raise your right leg. Raise it as far as you can and try to bring it around 90 degrees against the floor.

- Stay in this position for one minute and then slowly lower your leg.

- Repeat the step thrice.

- Next, practice the same with the left leg.

- Next, you should raise both the legs together. This can be a bit difficult initially. You might need to support your legs with your hands when you are doing it for the first time.

- Keep both the legs together and slowly raise them. Bring them at a distance of 90 degrees from the floor.

- Keep your legs in this position for 1 or 2 minutes before slowly lowering them back to the floor.

- This exercise helps in developing your abdominal muscles. It is also beneficial for your back.

- Keep your back straight and pressed against the floor while doing the entire series of leg raises.

2. Kapalbhati (Breathing Exercise).

- Kapalbhati is a popular form of breathing exercise in Yoga. It is a part of Pranayama. While practicing this exercise you should be relaxed and comfortable.

- Sit on the floor with your legs crossed.

- Keep your hands on your lap and slowly close your eyes.

- Start with a forceful exhale.
- Once you exhale forcefully, you will automatically inhale without any effort. Hence, all you have to concentrate on is to exhale forcefully.

- Keep on exhaling rapidly and forcefully. Continue doing this for as long as you can (begin with one minute.)

- When you are exhaling forcefully, your abdomen contracts. Every time you exhale your abdomen contracts inwards. And every time you inhale, your abdomen expands outwards automatically.

- Keep doing this for a minute. And once you stop, your breathing becomes very relaxed and very slow.

- This breathing exercise is quite beneficial in reducing the fat around the abdomen. It also aids in the development of abdominal muscles.

- It has several other benefits too. It helps in clearing the airways and it removes all the negative energy caught in your body.

- This exercise will help you in being more energetic and fresh. It can certainly help you in getting a 6-pack abs.

- During the initial stages you should perform this exercise for 1 minute. Eventually, you can increase the duration to 3 to 4 minutes. You can do this twice in a day.

3. Dhanurasana

- Dhanurasana is an important pose in Yoga which is quite popular for its long list of benefits. One of the most important benefits of doing this Asana is that it helps in reducing your stomach. It reduces the fat around the abdomen and makes it flat and fit.

- In Dhanurasana the body attains the shape of a bow. Dhanur is a Sanskrit term which means a 'bow'.

- To begin with this Asana you need to lie down on your belly.

- Reach out with your hands and try to hold your feet. Grab your feet by your ankles and raise your torso gently.

- Now your abdomen would be the only part that touches the ground.

- Stay in this position for a minute or two.

- This exercise is considered as one of the most effective yoga poses that helps in shaping your stomach.

- If you are trying to get a 6-pack abs then do this Asana twice daily. This will help you to carve your muscles without much difficulty.
- This Asana also aids in digestion. This in turn improves the absorption of nutrients and minerals.

4. Hastapadasana

- Hastapadasana is one of the basic Asanas or poses that helps in reducing weight.

- Stand erect and try to maintain a straight posture.

- Bend down and try to touch the floor with your hands.

- Keep your knees straight while you are bending.

- Keep your hands on the floor on either side of your feet.

- If it is difficult for you to place the hands on the floor, then try to touch your feet.

- Stay in this position for a minute.

- This Asana helps in reducing the fat around your belly.

- It helps in shaping and strengthening the muscles of your abdomen.

- It also strengthens the nervous system and this in turn will give you more energy to carry out your weight training and other workouts.

5. Paschimottanasana

- Paschimottanasana is quite similar to the last one we did.

- Sit on the floor keep your legs close to each other.

- Stretch your arms and reach for your feet.

- Bow down as far as you can and hold your feet with your hands.

- Stay in this position for a minute.

- This Asana helps in reducing the fat around the abdomen.

- Practice this Asana twice in a day to shape the muscles around your abdomen.

6. Naukasan

- Naukasan is a simple Asana and it can really help you if you are trying to reduce the fat around your abdomen.

- Lie on your belly and relax your entire body.

- Bring forward both your arms and extend them over your head.
- Join your hands in a prayer-like pose.

- Slowly lift your feet from the floor. Raise your legs as far as possible.

- Simultaneously raise your arms too. Along with your arms you should also raise your head and neck.

- Now your chest, abdomen and hips are the only parts that touch the ground.

- Stay in this position for a minute. Now your body resembles the shape of a boat. For this reason this Asana is known as Naukasana. Nauka is a Sanskrit word which means boat.

- This Asana helps in reducing the fat around your belly. It can definitely help you in developing a 6-pack abs.

7. Bhujangasana

- Lie on your belly and relax your whole body.

- With the support of your hands slowly raise your upper body.

- Raise your torso right from the stomach region.

- Turn your gaze upwards and remain still in this position.

- While doing this Asana your body acquires the shape of a snake that has spread its hood. The word Bhujanga means a snake.

- This Asana is also beneficial in shaping your abdomen and reducing the fat stores.

Along with your weight training and gym workouts, practice all the aforementioned yoga poses or Asanas to get a 6-pack abs.

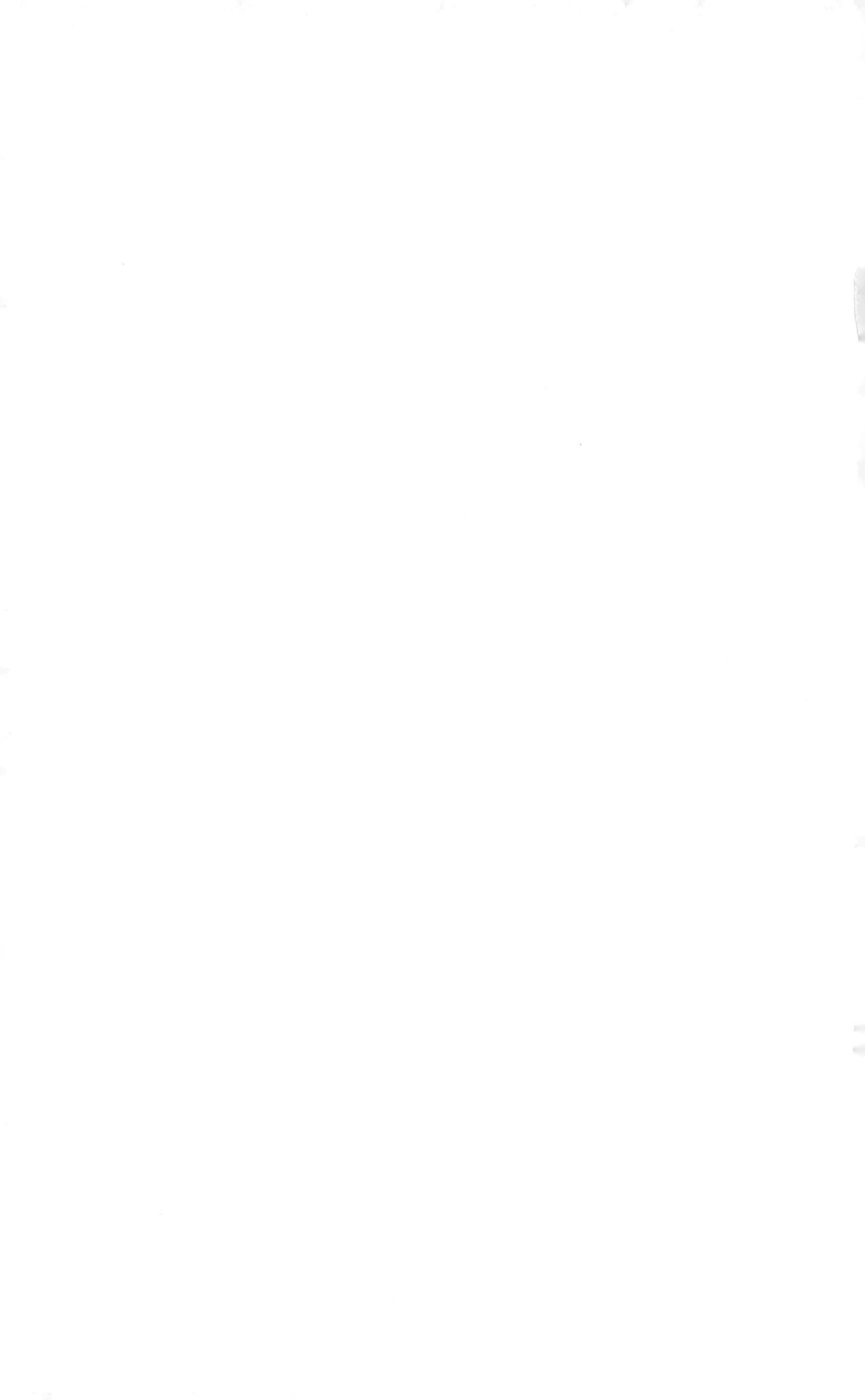

www.ingramcontent.com/pod-product-compliance
Lightning Source LLC
Chambersburg PA
CBHW072015280526
45788CB00005B/2053